HAPPY BIR

TO

....

WITH LOVE FROM

....

And Marilyn

HAPPY BIRTHDAY—LOVE . . .

Complete Series

Jane Austen

Joan Crawford

Bette Davis

Liam Gallagher

Audrey Hepburn

John Lennon

Bob Marley

Marilyn Monroe

Michelle Obama

Jackie Kennedy Onassis

Elvis Presley

Keith Richards

Frank Sinatra

Elizabeth Taylor

Oscar Wilde

HAPPY BIRTHDAY
Love, Marilyn

ON YOUR SPECIAL DAY

ENJOY THE WIT AND WISDOM OF

MARILYN MONROE

THE WORLD'S GREATEST STAR

Edited by Jade Riley

CELEBRATION BOOKS

THIS IS A CELEBRATION BOOK

Published by Celebration Books 2023
Celebration Books is an imprint of Dean Street Press

Text & Design Copyright © 2023 Celebration Books

All Rights Reserved. No part of this publication may be reproduced, stored in or transmitted in any form or by any means without the written permission of the copyright owner and the publisher of this book.

Cover by DSP

ISBN 978 1 915393 66 1

www.deanstreetpress.co.uk

HAPPY BIRTHDAY—LOVE, MARILYN

For countless fans, Marilyn Monroe is the quintessential Hollywood star and icon. It wasn't just her remarkable beauty and natural glamour that took her to the pinnacle of celebrity status. Maybe on the surface she possessed an image of blonde bombshell perfection, but it could never be said she was dumb. Conversely, she could never embody the ice princess because her humor and child-like sweetness spilled forth so easily from the screen. In fact, her warmth was so evident that many say she glowed with an inner light. In her numerous roles, she generated an approachability and kindness that made us all think she was also our friend.

During her own era, her acting talent was sadly underrated but in hindsight we realize she was never just "playing herself." In classic film roles she displayed a diversity that is often forgotten. Of course, we recall her in easy-to-love comedies such as the gold digging Lorelei Lee in *Gentlemen Prefer Blondes*, the ditzy model/upstairs neighbor in *The Seven Year Itch* and the vulnerable Cherie in *Bus Stop*. But look back to her femme fatale in *Niagara* or the heartbreaking Roslyn of *The Misfits*, as desperate to save the wild Mustang horses as she is to free

Clark Cable from his demons. Her acting range was wide, her complexity of character evident.

Let's not forget she could really sing and dance!

And so for your birthday, take a deep dive into Marilyn's own words. Celebrate life through this remarkable woman's point of view. The Beloved Legend, the Consummate Entertainer lived a rich life . . . so take a moment, close your eyes and imagine the silver screen goddess singing "Happy Birthday to you."

Marilyn Monroe

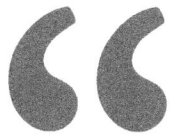

Nothing lasts forever, so live it up; drink it down, laugh it off, avoid the bullshit. Take chances and never have regrets because, at one point, everything you did was exactly what you wanted.

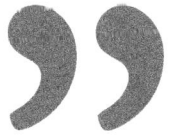

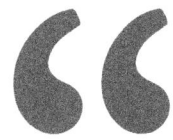

What do I wear in bed? Why, Chanel N° 5, of course.

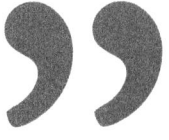

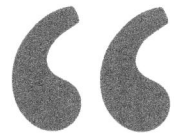

We are all of
us stars, and
we deserve to
twinkle.

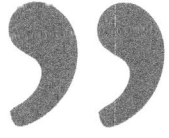

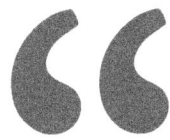

If I'd observed all the rules, I'd never have got anywhere.

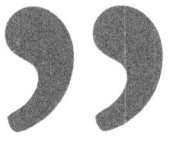

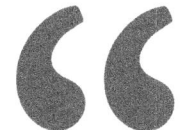

I
defy
gravity.

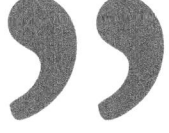

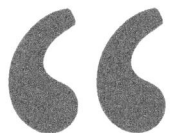

Keep smiling because life is a beautiful thing and there's so much to smile about.

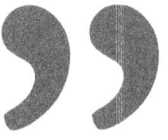

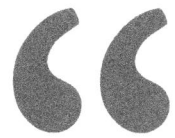

We should all start to live before we get too old.

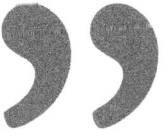

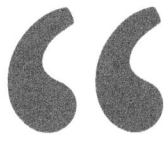

One of the best things that ever happened to me is that I'm a woman. That is the way all females should feel.

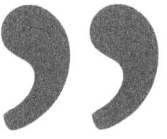

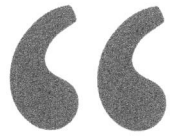

I want to grow old without facelifts. I want to have the courage to be loyal to the face I have made.

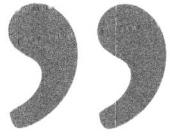

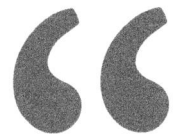

"I've been on a calendar, but I've never been on time.

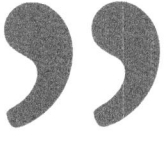
"

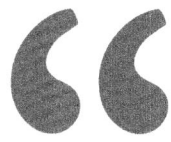

The body is meant to be seen, not all covered up.

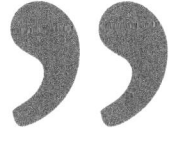

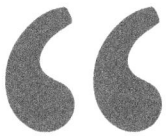

Imperfection is beauty, madness is genius and it's better to be absolutely ridiculous than absolutely boring.

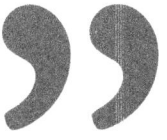

" Who said nights were for sleep? "

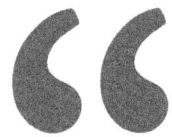

I'm very definitely a woman and I enjoy it.

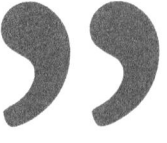

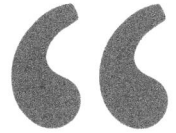

I like to feel blonde all over.

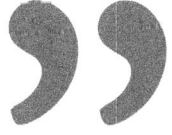

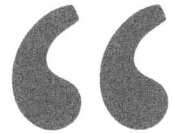

Dogs never bite me – just humans.

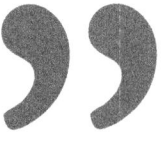

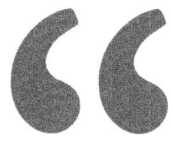

Give a girl the right shoes, and she can conquer the world.

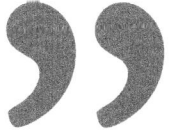

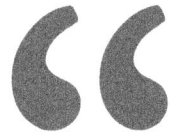

It's all make believe, isn't it?

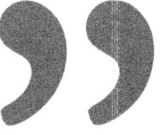

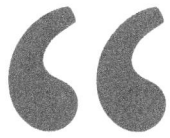

A smile is the best **makeup** a girl can wear.

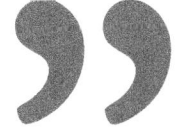

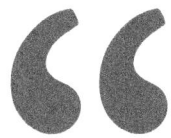

A wise girl knows her limits, a smart girl knows that she has none.

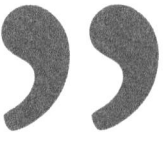

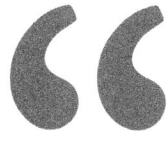

I don't mind living
in a man's world
as long as I can
be a woman in it.

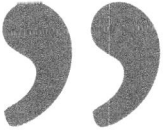

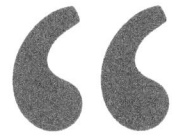

Always remember to smile and look up at what you got in life.

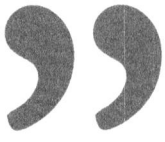

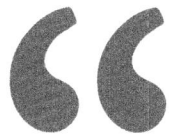

I learned to walk as a baby, and I haven't had a lesson since.

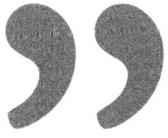

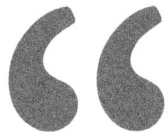

For those who are poor in happiness, each time is a first time; happiness never becomes a habit.

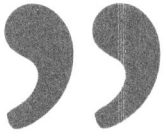

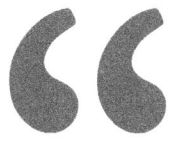

I don't know who invented high heels, but all women owe him a lot.

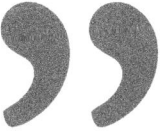

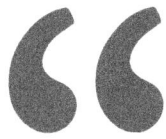

Confidentially, the type of male I find most enjoyable for a friend is one who has enough fire and assurance to speak up for his convictions.

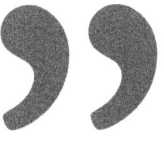

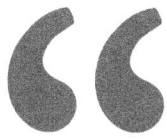

Experts on romance say for a happy marriage there has to be more than a passionate love. For a lasting union, they insist, there must be a genuine liking for each other. Which, in my book, is a good definition for friendship.

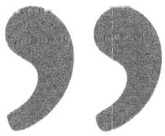

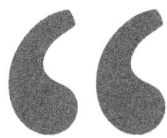

Success makes so many people hate you. I wish it wasn't that way. It would be wonderful to enjoy success without seeing envy in the eyes of those around you.

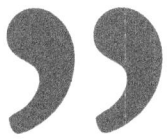

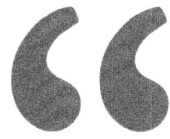

I don't want to make money.
I just want to be wonderful.

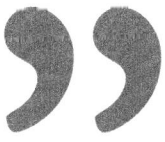

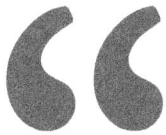

Fame is fickle, and I know it. It has its compensations but it also has its drawbacks, and I've experienced them both.

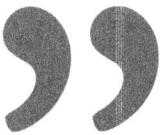

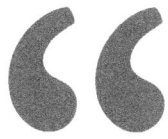

I think one of the basic reasons men make good friends is that they can make up their minds quickly.

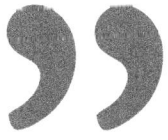

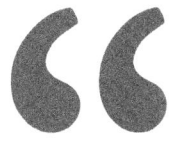

A friend tells you what you want to hear; a best friend tells you the truth.

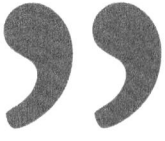

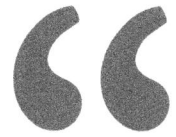

I read poetry to save time.

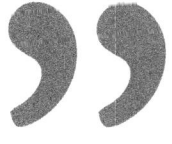

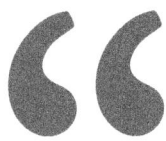

The real lover is the man who can thrill you just by touching your head or smiling into your eyes—or just by staring into space.

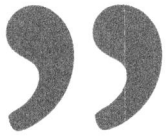

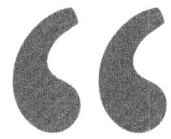

Sex is a part of nature. I go along with nature.

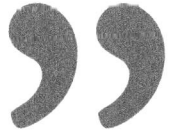

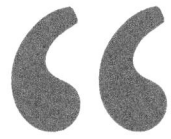

If you can make a girl laugh, you can make her do anything.

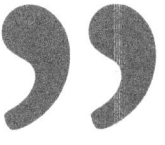

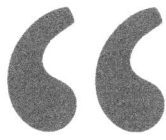

I don't forgive people because I'm weak, I forgive them because I am strong enough to know people make mistakes.

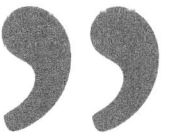

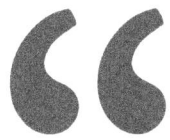

Fame is like caviar, you know—it's good to have caviar but not when you have it at every meal.

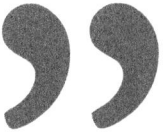

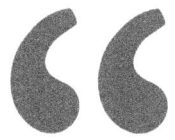

Fear is stupid.
So are regrets.

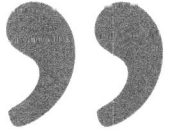

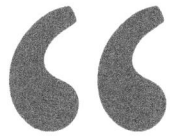

Sometimes good things fall apart so better things can fall together.

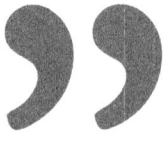

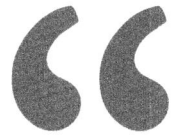

Dreaming about being an actress, is more exciting than being one.

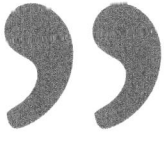

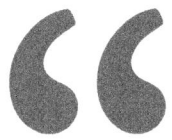

A career is born
in public—
talent in privacy.

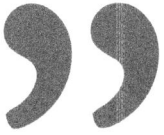

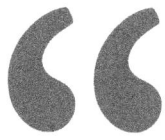

When it comes to gossip, I have to readily admit men are as guilty as women.

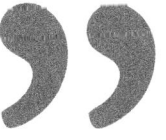

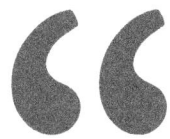

A career is wonderful, but you can't curl up with it on a cold night.

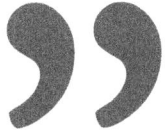

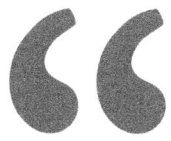

Millions of people live their entire lives without finding themselves. But it is something I must do.

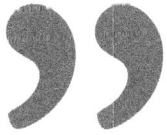

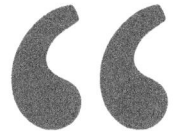

I restore myself when I'm alone.

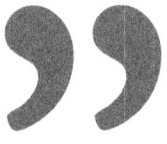

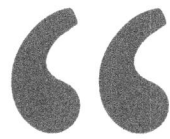

I don't understand why people aren't a little more generous with each other.

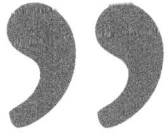

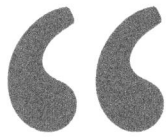

A woman knows by intuition, or instinct, what is best for herself.

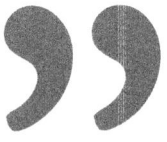

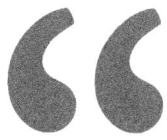

I'm selfish, impatient and a little insecure. I make mistakes, I'm out of control, and at times hard to handle. But if you can't handle me at my worst, then you don't deserve me at my best.

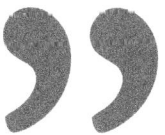

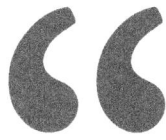

Hollywood is a place where they'll pay you a thousand dollars for a kiss and fifty cents for your soul.

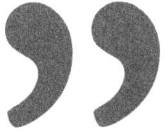

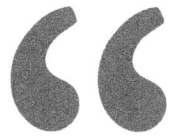

If you spend your life competing with business men, what do you have? A bank account and ulcers!

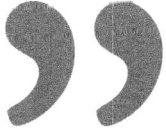

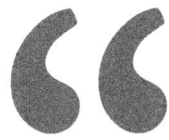

It was the creative part
that kept me going,
trying to be an actress.
I enjoy acting when
you really hit it right.

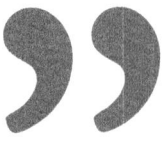

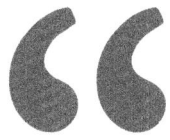

Designers want me to dress like spring, in billowing things. I don't feel like spring. I feel like a warm red autumn.

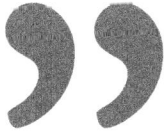

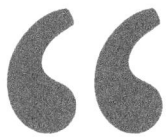

I think that we're rushing too much nowadays. That's why people are nervous and unhappy—with their lives and with themselves. How can you do anything perfect under such conditions?

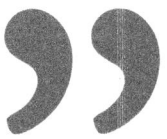

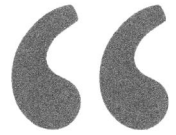

Perfection takes time.

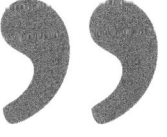

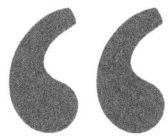

I think trying to be happy is almost as difficult as trying to be a good actress. You have to work at both of them.

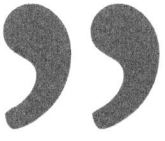

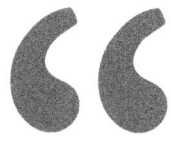

Love and work are the only things that really happen to us. Everything else doesn't really matter.

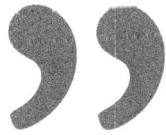

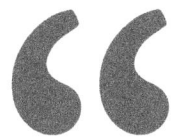

I'm not bored by things; I'm just bored by people who are bored.

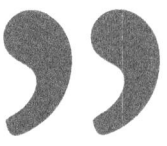

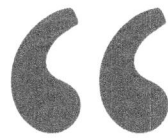

I can easily be alone and it doesn't bother me. I don't mind it—it's like a rest, it kind of refreshes myself.

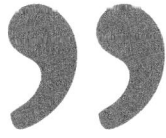

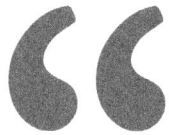

Men who think that a woman's past love affairs lessen her love for them are usually stupid and weak.

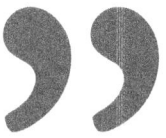

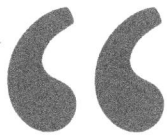

I don't think mankind was intended to be like machines. Besides, it's a great waste of time—you get more done doing it more sensibly, more leisurely.

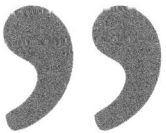

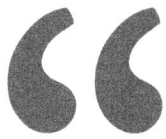

I am good, but not an angel. I do sin, but I am not the devil. I am just a small girl in a big world trying to find someone to love.

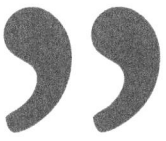

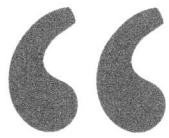

I knew I belonged to the public and to the world, not because I was talented or even beautiful, but because I had never belonged to anything or anyone else.

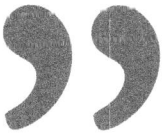

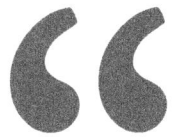

It's not true I had nothing on. I had the radio on.

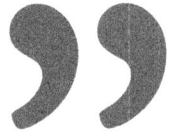

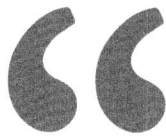

I never quite understood it, this sex symbol. I always thought symbols were those things you clash together! That's the trouble, a sex symbol becomes a thing.
I just hate to be a thing.

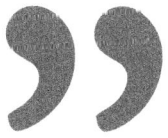

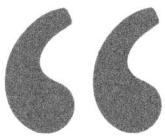

We are all born sexual creatures, thank God, but it's a pity so many people despise and crush this natural gift. Art, real art, comes from it, everything.

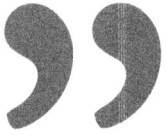

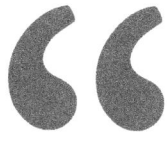

Your clothes should be tight enough to show you're a woman but loose enough to show you're a lady.

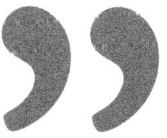

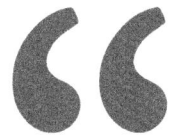

I like people.
The public
scares me, but
people I trust.

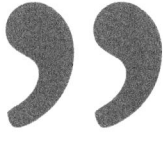

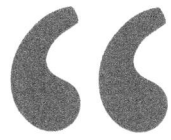

If there is only one thing in my life that I am proud of, it's that I've never been a kept woman.

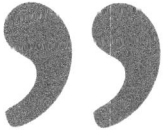

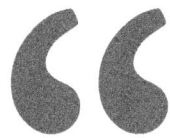

It might be a kind of relief to be finished. You have to start all over again. But I believe you're always as good as your potential.

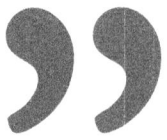

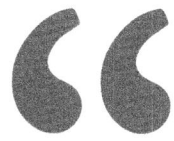

I'm trying to find the nailhead, not just strike the blow.

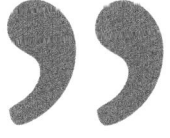

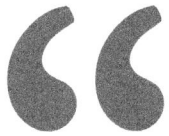

I don't think it would be very feminine to be tough. Guess I'll settle for the way I am.

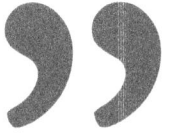

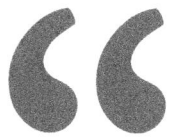

Every educated girl should know about the Essays of Montaigne.

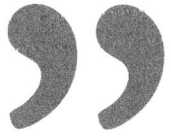

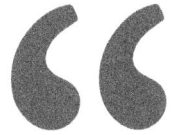

A smart girl leaves before she is left.

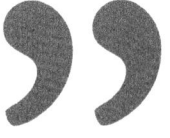

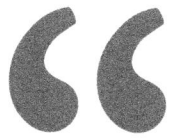

Fame doesn't fulfill you. It warms you a bit, but that warmth is temporary.

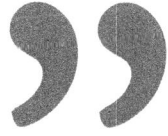

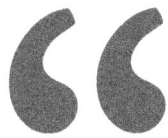

I have always had a talent for irritating women since I was fourteen.

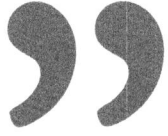

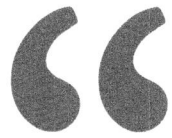

Friends accept you the way you are.

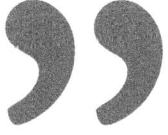

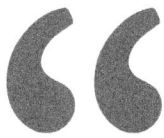

There is just no comparison between having a dinner date with a man and staying home playing canasta with the girls.

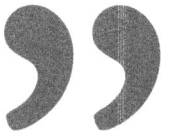

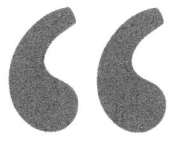

It is wonderful to have someone praise you, to be desired.

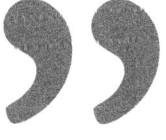

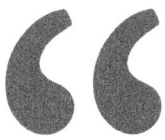

Sometimes I think it would be easier to avoid old age, to die young, but then you'd never complete your life, would you? You'd never wholly know you.

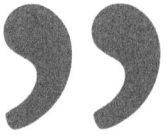

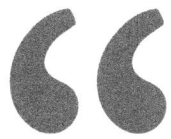

In Hollywood a girl's virtue is much less important than her hairdo.

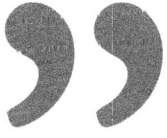

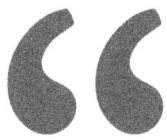

I like actors very much, but to marry one would be like marrying your brother. You look too much alike in the mirror.

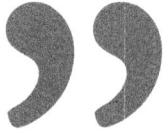

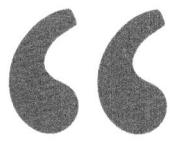

It's better to be unhappy alone than unhappy with someone—so far.

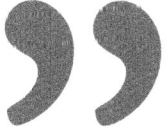

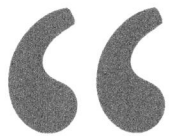

My popularity seems almost entirely a masculine phenomenon.

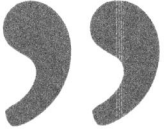

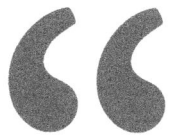

Always, always, always believe in yourself, because if you don't, then who will, sweetie?

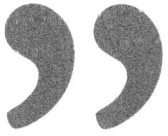

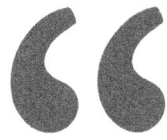

What good is it being Marilyn Monroe? Why can't I just be an ordinary woman?

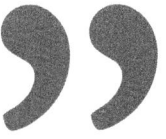

Marilyn Monroe

ABOUT THE EDITOR

Jade Riley is a writer whose interests include old movies, art history, vintage fashion and books, books, books.

Her dream is to move to London, to write like Virginia Woolf, and to meet a man like Mr. Darcy, who owns a vacation home in Greece.

Printed in Great Britain
by Amazon